a guide to womb discovery

22 WAYS TO HEAL HER

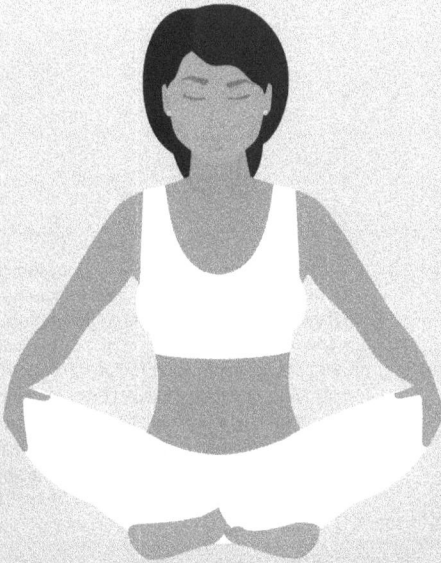

FELICIA GUY-LYNCH

Dedication

To all those striving to heal and maintain salvation

Believe

What are your values? Where do they come from?

check within

Forgive

Everyone is a villain in someone's story.
How can you heal the mind and body when you consciously
choose to nurse poison within your heart?

check out: theforgivenessproject.com

Abstain

You can't purge out if you keep letting the wrong energy in.
Is the right energy at the wrong time still the wrong energy?

check out: queenafua.com

Vent

The more you repress and suppress your emotions, the more
you stress out your womb.
Process.
Write it out.
Talk it out.
Repeat.

call a friend. meet up somewhere

Prognosis

Don't get into the trap of self-diagnosis.
Follow up.
Get a pelvic ultrasound.

call your doctor to book an appointment

Counseling

Get trusted, professional help to unpack, make sense of,
cope and overcome past trauma.
Healing Circles can help.

check out: therapyforblackgirls.com

Organic Pads

What are some benefits?

- Better for your body as they are free from dioxins (cancer-causing by-products of chlorine bleaching on conventional pads)
- Environmentally friendly as they are made from organic cotton
- Economically sustainable

check out: natracare.com

Yoni Pearls

What are they and why use them?
The herbal womb detox pearls have been specially created with ancient herbs that have been used for feminine wellness. They help combat bacteria vaginosis, foul odor, yeast infections, endometriosis and fibroids.

check out: embracepangaea.com

Womb Massage

What are some benefits?

- Helps to reposition a tilted uterus
- Promotes hormonal balance
- Breaks up scar tissue
- Brings fresh blood and circulation to the uterus and cervix
- Reduces stress & stress hormones
- Increases circulation to the uterus & cervix
- Encourages the liver to get rid of excess hormones
- Promotes hormonal balance by strengthening the hormonal feedback loop
- Assists in the purging of old stagnant blood and tissues

check out: thewomb.ca

Minerals

What are the benefits?

- Vitamins B Complex - helps to reduce menstrual cramps and moodiness
- Magnesium - helps to relieve menstrual cramps, help to alleviate irritability and anxiety
- Calcium - helps to reduce menstrual cramps, fluid retention and food cravings
- Zinc - helps to relieve menstrual cramps and depression
- Iron - helps to manage anemia

check out: thewomens.org.au

Enema

What's is it and the benefits?

- An enema is a procedure that involves injecting a liquid or gas, into the rectum through the anus to either administer medication or flush out fecal matter
- It can help with treating ulcerative colitis, alleviating severe constipation and assisting medical professionals with giving a diagnosis

check out: badgut.org

Exercise

What are the benefits to each workout?

- <u>Top Taps</u> are performed when you lie on your back with forearms at your sides, raise your feet off the floor to 90 degrees, lower your right leg to tap your toes on the floor, return to starting position then repeat with your left leg as you engage your core. This is beneficial because you utilize your abdominal muscles to help relieve cramps

- <u>The Seated Leg Forward Bend</u> brings relief to your lower back and sacrum, which can become tight and stiff during your period. First, you start in a seated position with your legs stretched out in front of you. On an exhale, slowly slide forward. Keep grounded as you lower your body toward legs and pull your stomach in to massage the lower abdomen. Hold, breathing deeply for 1 - 3 minutes, gently folding towards your legs

- <u>The Seated Twist</u> brings relief to the abdomen with a great massage to your entire back, where tension is often carried during this time of the month due to physical discomfort. You start in a seated position on the floor with your legs extended out in front of you. Bend your right knee and place your right foot near your left knee on the floor. Sit tall and flex the extended leg, then inhale, extending your left arm up towards the ceiling. Begin to rotate the spine towards the bent leg without lifting either hip from the floor. Work with this twist for 7 - 10 breaths. Repeat on the other side

check out: thehealthy.com

Ionic Foot Bath

What is it and the benefits?

- This process gives the hydrogen in the water a positive charge. The positive charge attracts the negatively charged toxins in your body. The ions in the foot bath water hold a charge that enables them to bind to heavy metals and toxins in your body. This allows the toxins to be pulled out through the bottoms of your feet
- It can help with reducing menstrual cramps, menopause symptoms, sexual health problems, acne, restlessness, stress and yeast infections

Color of the Water	Area of the Body Represented/Detoxified
Black	liver
Black Flecks	heavy metals
Blue	kidney
Brown	liver, tobacco, cellular debris
Green	gallbladder
Orange	joints
Red Flecks	cellular debris, blood clot material
Yellow	kidney, bladder, urinary tract, female/prostate area
Cheesy	candidas, fungal infections, most likely yeast
Foam	lymphatic drainage, mucus
Oil Floating	fat

Natural Progesterone

What are some benefits?
- Treats infertility by helping the uterine line to become thick enough for successful implantation
- Maintain pregnancy to prevent miscarriage
- Boosts low progesterone levels in women who have polycystic ovarian syndrome (PCOS)
- Alleviates menopausal symptoms such as hot flashes, sleeplessness and low bone density

Red Clover

What are some benefits?
- Support proper lymphatic function
- Immune support
- Aids in healthy skin
- Used a tonic for menstrual irregularity and menopause

check out: gaiaherbs.com

Lemon and Ginger

What are some benefits?

- Fights infection with its combined anti-inflammatory, anti-bacterial, anti-fungal, anti-diabetic, anti-cancer and anti-viral properties
- Reduces nausea
- Optimizes thyroid health

check out: emilykylenutrition.com

Bentonite Clay and Psyllium Husk

consult a health professional

What are some benefits?

The bentonite clay absorbs toxins and the psyllium husk scrubs out the corners of your intestines. This encourages the:

- Removal of plastics and heavy metals
- Reversal of radiation exposure
- Alleviation of symptoms associated with irritable bowel syndrome (IBS)

Grounded
Flaxseed

What are some benefits?
- Protects the brain with omega-3 fatty acids
- Protects the heart with linoleic acid
- Aids the body in flushing out extra estrogen

check out: womenshealthmag.com

Colon
Hydrotherapy

It is commonly referred to as a colonic irrigation or colon cleansing. It's similar to an enema but uses more liquid along with special herbs, enzymes or probiotics to accentuate the healing process.

Some of the benefits are that it stimulates bowel movement, increases your chances of fertility and helps to maintain a healthy pH level for your blood.

check out: yurielkaim.com

Fiber Intake

What are the different types?

Cellulose - insoluble fiber found in vegetables like cabbage that bind to other food particles to assist with bowel movement

Inulin - soluble fiber derived from chicory root found naturally in wheat like barley. It leaves you feeling fuller for longer by slowing down digestion

Pectin - soluble fiber found in vegetables like strawberries helps reduce the glycemic response of foods by stalling glucose absorption. In other words, no sugar spikes

Beta-Glucans - a gel-forming type of soluble fiber found in foods like reishi mushrooms that easily gets broken down by the gut flora

Psyllium - a prebiotic, soluble fiber found in high-fiber cereals that help relieve constipation by softening bowels to help it pass

Lignin - an insoluble fiber that's part of the cell wall structure in plants such as avocados that may help to reduce the risk of developing colon cancer

Resistant Starch - a type of fiber found in legumes and beans that passes through the large intestine, protecting the GI tract from harmful bacteria

Overall, fiber helps your liver and digestive system to remove and eliminate excess estrogen.

Fermented Foods

What are the different types?

Lactic Acid Fermentation - relies on yeasts and bacteria to convert starches and sugars into lactic acid and contains live organisms (probiotics) E.g.) <u>Sauerkraut, kombucha, kimchi and bread</u>

Ethyl Alcohol Fermentation - uses yeast to break down starches and sugars to make <u>wine and beer</u> but does not contain live organisms

Acetic Acid Fermentation - vinegar is used to make fermented foods such as <u>pickles</u>

Overall, fermented foods protect the intestinal mucous membrane from leaking, alleviates symptoms in autoimmune disorders and plays a key role in helping your body maintain a healthy gut-brain relationship.

check out: mindbodygreen.com

Epsom Salt Bath

The two main ingredients of Epsom salt are magnesium and sulfate. The two combined stimulate detoxification.

Magnesium aids in the body's ability to remove toxins responsible for inflammation while also reducing swelling, stiffness and pain.

Sulfate can strengthen the walls of the digestive tract and make releasing toxins easier.

Adding therapeutic oils such as lavender can make a detox bath more relaxing.

source: medicalnewstoday.com